Ski Shape

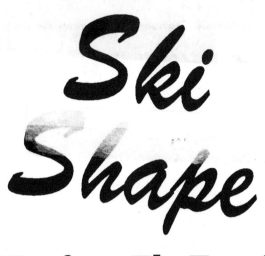

How To Get Fit For Skiing
The Ultimate Illustrated Guide

Designed and Edited by Hal Schuster

Ski Shape

How To Get Fit For Skiing
The Ultimate Illustrated Guide

David Lessnick

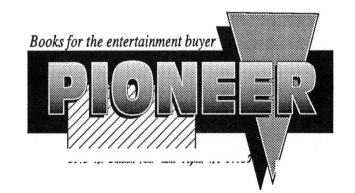

Books for the entertainment buyer

PIONEER

ADDITIONAL CREDITS

Front cover photography, Vino Anthony (large shot), Stephanie Brignone (inserts)

Back cover photography, Vino Anthony

Inside photography, Emily Fishman

Female models, Stephanie Rene and Chris Wilson

Library of Congress Cataloging-in-Publication Data
David Lessnick, 1966—
    SKI SHAPE: How to Get Fit for Skiing

    1.   SKI SHAPE: How to Get Fit for Skiing (fitness)
I. Title

Published by Pioneer Books, Inc., 5715 N. Balsam Rd., Las Vegas, NV, 89130.

First Printing, 1992

Dedicated To Adam and Lindsay

There is so much involved in putting a book of this nature together.

My special thanks go to John Atkins, Frank Salgado, and Dr. Bob Hintermeister. The manuscript is as complete and correct as it is because of their expertise, time, and encouragement. Of course, what is not correct is my own.

I also want to thank my publisher, Has Schuster, for helping an idea become a reality. There was a great amount of work pulling this book together and Hal did not settle for any shortcuts.

I am also greatful to Vino Anthony, Stephanie Brignone, and Emily Fishman for their time and great pictures and to Chris Wilson and Stephanie Rene for their time and beauty.

Of course, the acknowledgements wouldn't be complete without a special thanks to my mom. All my accomplishments are hers because she is always there in all the right ways.

ABOUT THE AUTHOR

DAVID LESSNICK is a professionally certified ski instructor (PSIA) and has been involved with skiing since the age of four. He lives part time in Colorado and teaches all levels of skiing at Vail/Beaver Creek. David has an extensive background in gymnastics both as a competitor and coach. He was the Nevada State Champion and later coached for one of the top boys programs in the country where he was in charge of strength/conditioning training. When he's not in Vail, he lives in Las Vegas where he teaches a SKI SHAPE class and runs a marketing company.

ABOUT THIS BOOK

SKI SHAPE: HOW TO GET FIT FOR SKIING is really a first of its kind. I wrote this book because many of my students were asking me (and other instructors told me the same) what they could do, or should do, to get in shape for skiing. They said that outside of a few articles in ski magazines, there was no help available.

I quickly discovered this was the sad truth. The few books I found are so outdated that many of the exercises they suggest have proved more harmful than beneficial. A lot of people—and obviously your one of them since you're reading this—want to get the most out of skiing, and preparing physically is a good start.

SKI SHAPE: HOW TO GET FIT FOR SKIING is written with the idea that most people lead extremely busy lifestyles and demand the most from their time. If you follow the program in this book, you will improve your SKI SHAPE an your skiing in just two hours a week

Each exercise tells you which muscles are trained and the exact "ski specific" benefits. There are three different 12 week training programs ranging from beginner to advanced to get you started and keep you on track.If you follow the exercises, you wil ski with more confidence and enjoyment than ever before.

—David Lessnick

FOREWORD

David Lessnick's SKI SHAPE is a winner! This Book not only gives any level of skier the proven basic exercises, but also many of the latest "secret" world cup exercises. David leads you through a realistic goal setting to the fitness precautions of getting a doctors O.K. and finally how to hook up with a knowledgeable trainer for the more advanced exercises. David has enlisted the help of Mike Farney, one of the best athletes to ever ski for the U.S. Ski Team. Mike adds years of World Cup experience to a great new ski shape program. Good luck guys!

Sincerely,
John Atkins MS-A.T.C.

13   INTRODUCTION

17   WHY TRAIN?

21   ANALYZING A SKIERS NEEDS

27   SETTING GOALS

31   COMPONENTS OF A SKI SPECIFIC WORK OUT

35   WARM-UP EXERCISES

39   STRETCHING

49   AEROBIC AND ANAEROBIC

55   SKI SPECIFIC WEIGHT TRAINING

67   SKI SPECIFIC POWER TRAINING

73   SKI SPECIFIC CROSS TRAINING

79   TRAINING PROGRAM

85   ON SNOW WARM-UP

91 HOME WORK OUT

99 SKIING SKILLS

103 ENERGY FOODS FOR SKIING

109 ASSESSING SKIING LEVEL

113 FINDING A TRAINER

117 YOUR PERSONAL TRAINING CHARTS

120 SKIIER'S RESPONSIBILITY CODE

SKI SHAPE: How To Get Fit for Skiing

12 SKI SHAPE

INTRODUCTION

I've skied for a very long time both as a member of the U.S. Ski Team and a coach for the University of Colorado's Ski Team. In the world of competitive skiing, the element that separates the winners from the rest of the pack is physical conditioning.

Here's the thing. . . physical conditioning is even more important for the recreational skier! Nothing will hinder your skiing more than being out of ski shape. David Lessnick has done a wonderful job in putting together realistic training programs that are very ski specific. He shows you not only how to get the most out of each exercise, but how to have fun while doing them. David is a great skier who loves the sport and blends his extensive gymnastics background with his knowledge of skiing in SKI SHAPE.It is written in a straight forward, easy to understand fashion and is perfect for the beginning athlete or the advanced expert.

By following the simple exercises in this book you will most certainly be skiing at a higher level with less chance of injury and with more enjoyment than you ever thought possible.

**Mike Farny,
Member U.S. Ski Team 1983-1986,
currently appearing in Warren Miller
Ski Films**

16 SKI SHAPE

1 WHY TRAIN?

" If you do what you've always done, you'll get what you've always gotten." -Anonymous

We have all felt it before. . . legs burning like a five alarm fire, lungs screaming for relief, mind and body acting not as one but as bitter enemies. . . and that's after only the first ski run of the day! O.K., so maybe I'm exaggerating a bit, but if you're like the majority of recreational skiers, you are not in good SKI SHAPE.

As a private ski instructor at Vail/Beaver Creek, I always ask my clients what their goals for their lessons are. Typical responses include: "skiing the bumps without getting any," "floating through the powder," or simply "skiing with more control and confidence." As a responsible instructor, I try to assess their fitness level by asking what they have done to get in shape for the ski season. At this point, I usually get a blank stare accompanied by a look of guilt. You know, the same look you used to give your parents when they asked what happened to the last piece of cake.

You've spent a year planning your ski trip, making countless reservations, reading all the consumer reports, and buying all new equipment. You've traveled hundreds of miles to your destination and spent untold dollars. Just imagine the cobalt blue skies, magnificent snow-covered peaks, and fresh mountain air. You've worked hard to make this trip a reality, but are you ready to ski?

To get in shape most people drive to the video store, rent a Warren Miller or Gregg Stump ski movie, and pop it into the VCR. Some jog a few miles a week or do sporadic weight training. Many convince themselves they can ski into shape.

Ask yourself, what *you* have done in the way of "ski specific" training. That is, what you have done to exercise not only the specific muscles used in skiing, but in the same way you will use them. Only "ski specific" training will get you in SKI SHAPE.

Think about it for a second. What other sport allows you to attain speeds of thirty miles per hour (without a motor), carry two hundred pounds of pressure on one leg, and balance on two long boards with your feet encased in heavy plastic boots?

Whether you are a ski racer on the slopes two hundred days a year or a weekend warrior in heaven if you ski ten days, you need "ski specific" training to get you in SKI SHAPE. You need this training for three reasons: 1) to reduce injuries; 2) to increase performance; and, 3) to make skiing more enjoyable.

According to the National Ski Patrol's Bruce Bacca, most ski injuries are fatigue-related and can be avoided through proper conditioning. "Skiing into shape does not work," added Bacca.

Few people ski a hundred days a year. Only if you begin in shape can you increase your performance within the few days you do ski. Otherwise you spend too much time regaining last year's skills.

Remember the last time you took a test? Did you do better going in cold turkey or when you prepared for it by studying in a "test specific" manner? If you want to increase performance, you need to train in "ski specific" ways. (Getting the hint yet?)

If you train properly, when your moment of truth on the slopes comes, you'll have the ability and confidence to perform your best.

"Ski specific" training will make you feel lighter on your skis. You will be more powerful and agile, quicker, and less easily fatigued. You will feel like a lean, mean, skiing machine ready for the steepest faces, toughest bumps, and narrowest chutes. Even a beginner will learn the sport more quickly and with greater ease because of "ski specific" training. "Ski specific" training means confidence, enjoyment, and a safer experience on the slopes for *you*!

2 ANALYZING A SKIERS NEEDS . . .

" Don't find fault, find a remedy." -Henry Ford

Before you start your training program it is important to understand the major physiological components involved in skiing and the terms used to describe them. Don't worry, I'm going to keep this simple and straightforward. Let's start with a list from which we will build a "ski specific" training program. I will then explain each component.

1. BODY AWARENESS
2. FLEXIBILITY
3. AEROBIC CAPACITY
4. ANAEROBIC CAPACITY
5. MUSCLE ENDURANCE
6. MUSCLE STRENGTH
7. POWER
8. COORDINATION

9. BALANCE
10. AGILITY
11. QUICKNESS

BODY AWARENESS

Body awareness is the ability to know where your body (or parts of your body) is in space without looking at it. For example, if you're in the dark and reach out with your hand, you know where it is even though you can't see it. You also know where your feet are even though you can't always see them. In skiing your body constantly changes position and body awareness allows you to keep track of it.

FLEXIBILITY

Flexibility is measured by the range of motion of the limbs about a particular joint, and by the elasticity of ligaments, tendons, and muscles surrounding that joint. Good flexibility can be achieved through proper stretching.

As a skier, you are frequently off balance. Body awareness coupled with greater flexibility will help you recover balance, greatly reducing the risk of muscle pulls and tears.

AEROBIC CAPACITY

Aerobic training involves low intensity, long duration activity (minimum of twenty minutes). It improves your body's ability to utilize oxygen so that your muscles won't fatigue as quickly. Although skiing is more anaerobic than aerobic (when was the last time you skied twenty minutes non-stop?), you may need to improve your aerobic capacity to do many of the exercises outlined in this book. Good aerobic capacity will also help you to enjoy a full day of skiing.

To build aerobic capacity you must find your ideal training range. Ideal training range is the number of heart beats per minute that must be sustained for a minimum of twenty minutes. Find your ideal training range by subtracting your age from 220 and multiplying by a number between .60 and .85, depending on your current aerobic capacity.

For example, a 35-year-old skier who already has been doing aerobics a few times a week will subtract 35 from 220 and multiply that number by .75 for a total of 139 heartbeats per minute. Once this skier reaches his target range of heartbeats per minute, that level of exercise must be maintained for at least twenty minutes.

ANAEROBIC CAPACITY

Anaerobic capacity refers to your ability to perform a maximum effort for relatively short duration without adequate oxygen being supplied to the muscles. Think of the last time you sprinted all out to catch a plane to your favorite ski resort. In skiing short turns are anaerobic; long turns are aerobic. Increase your anaerobic capacity and you will make better short turns—it really is that simple.

MUSCLE ENDURANCE

This is when a muscle or group of muscles work against a moderate resistance over an extended period of time without undue fatigue. If you have ever taken a long "cruiser run" followed by an even longer break in the lodge rubbing out a cramp, you know why muscular endurance is a must for skiing! Don't be a rubber-legged skier. Work on muscle endurance and get the most out of your day.

MUSCLE STRENGTH

Muscle Strength is the ability to exert a force. This is probably the single most important factor in skiing and all other athletic performance. Strength is measured by a muscle or group of mucles moving a mass a given distance. It is the foundation of muscle endurance, power, coordination, balance, agility, and quickness. If you want to hold an edge better, get stronger.

POWER

Power is a combination of strength and speed when time is an important factor. Short turns involve quick and decisive pressure on the edges of the skis. This requires power generated from the hips and legs.

COORDINATION

Everything we do requires some level of coordination. Coordination is the ability to perform a skilled movement pattern. Some of us were born with a natural sense of coordination; others still have a hard time walking without falling. Skiing requires a great deal of coordination blending steering, pressure, and edging skills. Fear not, stick to the SKI SHAPE program and you will be doing things you never thought you could.

BALANCE

The ability to maintain equilibrium as your body changes position is balance. Skiing is very dynamic. In one turn you can go from loose powder to groomed snow to ice. If you don't readjust your balance with each change, you will truley be "one with the snow."

AGILITY

Agility is closely related to coordination, strength, and balance. It is the ability to change direction with *quickness* while maintaining balance and coordination. Have you ever seen someone make a miraculous recovery?—that was agility!

QUICKNESS

Quickness is measured by the amount of time it takes to start a movement and how long it takes to finish the movement once started. Remember, skiing is a dynamic sport in which forces of nature test your ability to react instantaneously. If you aspire to ski the trees, you will need to be quick.

3 SETTING GOALS

" For every disiplined effort there is a multiple reward."- Jim Rohn

How many times do you start something with all the best intentions and get sidetracked.

Setting proper training goals can make or break your SKI SHAPE program. If you want to accomplish something, you need to set goals. Don't go into the gym or hop on your bike unless you have something specific you want to accomplish. If each exercise you complete brings you closer to your goal, you will be more motivated. For example, if your SKI SHAPE program prepares you to have more fun on the slope, you will work harder towards your goal.

If you write down your goals, and look at them each day, you will have a greater chance of reaching them.

Goals should be **S*M*A*R*T**:

*SPECIFIC—the goal you are you trying to accomplish

*MEASURABLE—the distance travelled toward your goal

*ATTAINABLE—keeping your goal realistic

*RELEVANT—the reason for the goal

*TRACKABLE—over a period of time

Here's an example of a **S*M*A*R*T** training goal: Every Monday at 6am I will do 25 push-ups and 50 sit-ups to help me become a better skiier..

KEEP TRAINING FUN

Riding my mountain bike in the crisp cool morning or skating on my Rollerblades as the sun drops behind the horizon gives me a sense of spiritual elation and overwhelming peacefulness. On my rugged bike I pedal hard as I jump over obstacles and negotiate the challenging terrain. With my Rollerblades I sprint up hills as hard as I can, knowing that once at the top, I can glide down making ski turns. This is too much fun. Can it actually be training?

The secret to a good training program that you will stick to is to keep the exercises fun and challenging. Then you will have too much fun to think about the burning sensation in your muscles or your shortness of breath. After all, if you enjoy what you are doing, you will do it longer, harder, with more motivation, and want to do it again the very next day. Fortunately, many exercises and activities that are great for skiing are also fun.

This book will give you exercises and cross training activities specific to skiing. Comprehensive SKI SHAPE programs are offered for the beginner, intermediate, and expert skier. Please make these your programs. Use what you like and don't worry about the rest. Train hard, be creative in your training, and you will enjoy your skiing as never before.

4 COMPONENTS OF A *SKI SPECIFIC* WORKOUT

*" Our bodies are our gardens. . . our will our gardeners." -
William Shakespeare*

Your SKI SHAPE workout will be broken down into four parts:

1. warm up
2. stretching
3. main workout
4. cool down

WARM UP

It is a common mistake to stretch before warming up. Stretching a "cold" muscle tears it down without increasing elasticity. It's like gunning your car engine before the oil lubricates the parts. A good warm up stimulates blood flow by increasing internal temperature and gets your body in a *ready* state by making tendons, ligaments, and muscles more pliable.

STRETCHING

Stretching increases your flexibility and gives your muscles greater resiliency. Well-stretched muscles better absorb changes in terrain and lessen the chances of pulls and tears when your limbs get in extreme ranges of motion.

MAIN WORKOUT

The main workout can consist of aerobics, anaerobics, weight training, power training, ski related activities (cross training), or a combination of the four.

COOL DOWN

During the main workout lactic acid builds up in the muscles causing stiffness and soreness the next day. The cool down period consists of stretching to retain flexibility after your muscles have been contracting (constantly shortening). Performing simple, relaxed motions with the body parts trained will increase circulation and aid in removing lactic acid and bringing fresh nutrients (metabolites) to the muscles. A proper cool down may shorten recuperation time. It is the most effective time to stretch!

WARNING: Before beginning any exercise program, consult with your physician. If you experience pain, shortness of breath or dizziness, stop exercising and call a physician.

5

WARM-UP EXERCISES

"Our doubts are traitors, And make us lose the good we oft might win, By fearing to attempt."—William Shakespeare

Warm-up exercises should be done on a soft surface to avoid unnecessary stress to the joints and should be performed for a minimum of five minutes non-stop.

JUMPING JACKS

Jumping jacks have been around for a long time for a good reason. . . they work! Start with your feet together and arms at your side. In one motion, bring your arms up until your hands touch and, at the same time, jump to a straddle with your legs about shoulder width apart. Land with your knees slightly bent. Then jump back to the starting position. Do these on a soft surface such as grass, a mat, or carpeting for about five minutes.

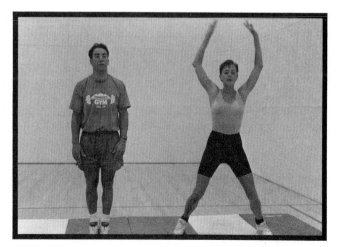

JUMP ROPE

If you are a little more aggressive, you can jump rope. This is an excellent "ski specific" warm-up because it promotes eye-foot coordination as you jump over the moving rope. Start out at a comfortable pace and then increase the speed. To make the exercise "ski specific", jump lateraly from foot to foot. Longer, slower jumps simulate long turns while short, fast jumps simulate short turns. Do these on a soft surface such as grass, a mat, or carpeting. Land with your knees slightly bent. Remember, if you look straight ahead instead of at your feet, you will increase your coordination and body awareness.

At left: Basic Jump
At right: The more advanced Lateral Jump

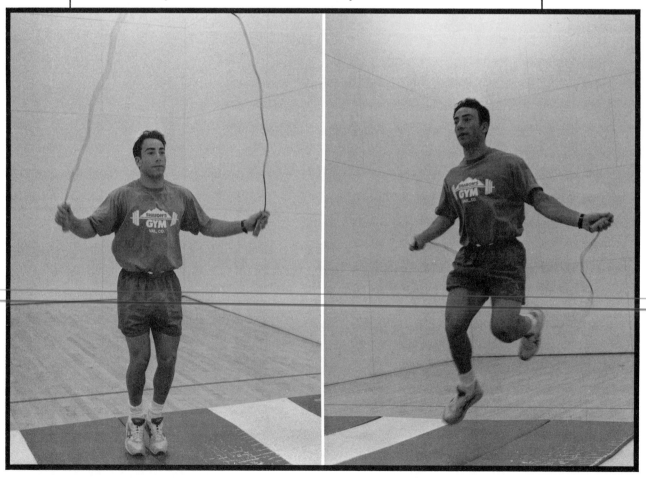

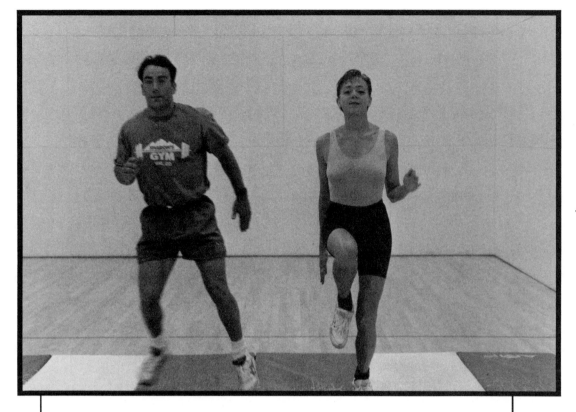

Keep your upper body still and always look forward

RUNNING IN PLACE

This is an easy warm-up, but don't cheat yourself. Make sure you get those legs and arms pumping to ensure blood flow.

SKI SPECIFIC BENEFITS
Promotes eye-foot coordination
Increases turning power

WARNING: Before beginning any exercise program, consult with your physician. If you experience pain, shortness of breath or dizziness, stop exercising and call a physician.

6 STRETCHING

"Don't find fault, find a remedy."-Henry Ford

I f you don't stretch properly you can injure yourself. While stretching is an important activity, it is crucial that it be done in the proper way to avoid unnecessary injuries. The four forms of stretching are: 1) ballistic, 2) static, 3) dynamic, and 4) partner resistance.

BALLISTIC STRETCHING

Ballistic stretching involves bouncing movement with no 'hold' as you go through the range of motion. It is widely agreed that ballistic stretching involves an inherent danger of overstraining connective tissue and should be avoided. As a gymnast, I have spent hundreds of hours stretching and recommend you avoid ballistic movements.

STATIC STRETCHING

Static stretching involves stretching until resistance is felt, stretching just beyond this point, and holding for twenty to thirty seconds.

Some do's and don'ts of static stretching:

1. only stretch when muscles are warm

2. avoid jerky movements

3. keep legs straight in straddle (legs apart) and pike (legs together) positions

4. begin 'hold' period as you feel resistance and increase the range as resistance subsides

5. breathe in deeply and exhale slowly at 'holding' point.

6. the no pain no gain theory does not apply—if you are in pain, you are probably tearing the muscle, not stretching it

DYNAMIC STRETCHING

Dynamic stretching is quickly becoming popular and is highly recommended by physical therapists and sports trainers. The method involves continuing movements that stretch muscles in a specific way. Since skiing is a dynamic sport, this type of stretching is very appropriate. Running in place with your knees lifted high is an example of a dynamic stretch.

PARTNER RESISTANCE STRETCHING

Partner resistance stretching adds the benefit of a partner applying resistance. While there are many advantages of stretching with a partner, it is imperative that each partner be knowledgeable and use safe techniques. The major advantage of partner resistance stretching is that it can increase your flexibility more quickly than stretching alone. Your partner can apply resistance (isometric resistance), fatiguing the muscle, allowing you to stretch further.

This is an advanced form of stretching that is dangerous if not done properly. You must communicate with your partner so he or she knows how much resistance to apply.

STRETCHING EXERCISES

The major muscle groups you need to stretch for skiing are: hamstrings (back of upper legs), quadriceps (front of upper legs), adductors (inner thigh), and abductors (outer thigh). Other muscle regions include calves, shins, back, neck, and shoulders.

HAMSTRING STRETCHES

be sure to keep your back straight when performing the following two stretches1.

PIKE

*in seated position place legs straight out in front and keep knees locked

*grab ankles and pull chest to knees

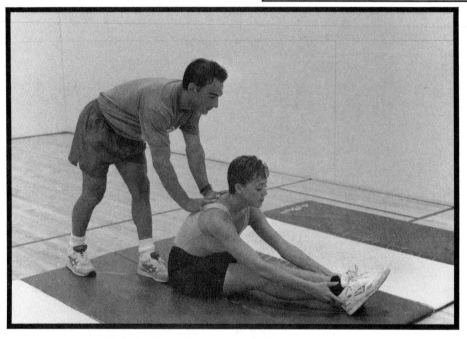

TOP: Pike Stretch with Partner Resistance

BOTTOM: Keep back straight and reach out to toes while

STRADDLE

*straddle as wide as comfortable in seated position

*reach both hands to one foot and pull chest towards knee (repeat with other side)

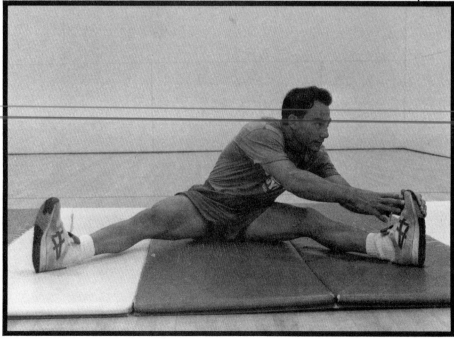

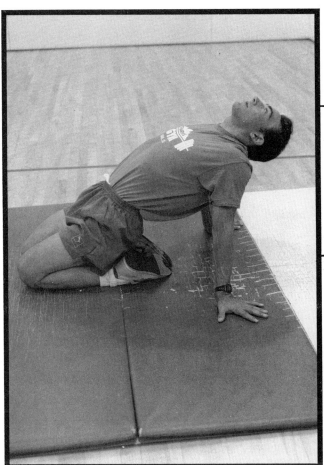

**QUADRICEPS
STRETCHES**

KNEE BENDER

*sitting on knees, sit back until seat touches heels.

*place hands on floor for balance stretching backwards keeping seat on heels.

PELICAN

*standing, lift one heel towards seat and grab ankle with hand

*pull foot towards seat and pull knee back and up

(you may need to hold on to something for balance but work towards doing it with no assistance as this will help your balance for skiing!)

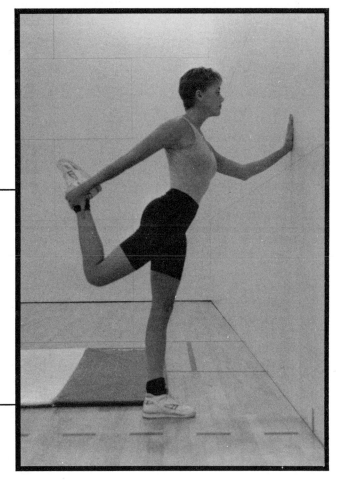

ADDUCTOR STRETCHES

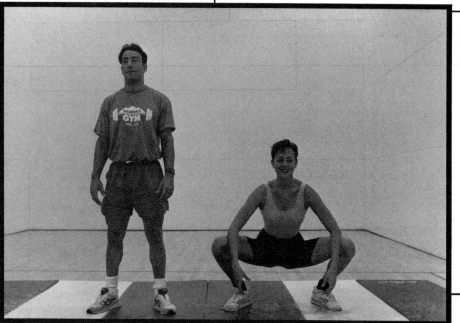

SUMO

*standing, place feet pointed outward and wider than shoulders.

*keeping heels on ground and back straight, sink down to 90 degree angle with knees.

*place elbows on inside of knees and press outwards

CHICKEN WING

*sitting, place soles of feet together and with hands, draw heels close to seat.

*using elbows, press outwards on knees towards ground

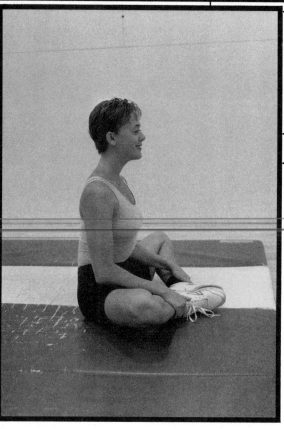

ABDUCTOR STRETCH

SINGLE KNEE

*laying on back, pull one knee towards opposite shoulder (repeat with other knee)

CALF STRETCH

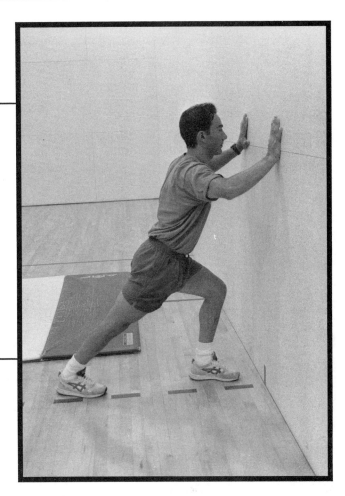

WALL HOLDS

*facing a wall, stand about two feet from it, place feet shoulder width apart

*keeping heels on floor and arms straight, reach out placing hands on wall

*bend arms bringing face close to wall (applying upward pressure against wall with palms will increase your stretch)

BACK STRETCH

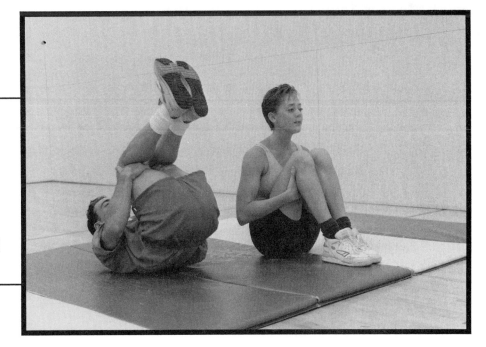

TUCK

*laying on back, bring both knees to chest

*pull knees in tight with hands and rock back and forth

SHOULDER STRETCH

FAR REACH

*sitting on floor in pike, place hands on floor behind you pointing fingers away from back

*without moving hands, walk feet and seat away from hands

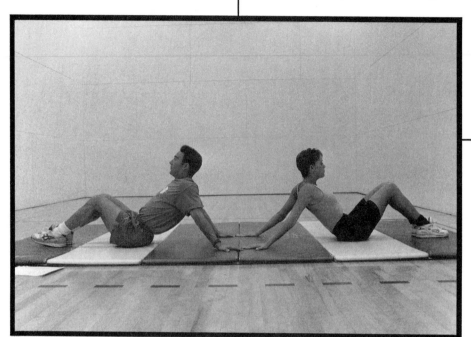

NECK STRETCH

FOUR POINTS

*pull chin to chest and hold

*touch left ear to left shoulder and hold

*touch right ear to right shoulder and hold

*look up at ceiling and hold

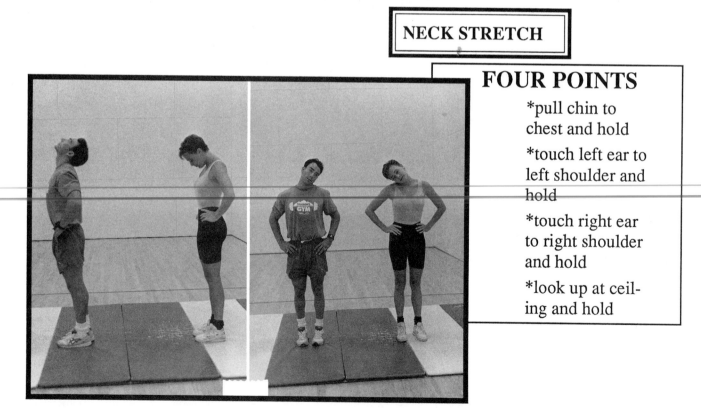

WARNING: Before beginning any exercise program, consult with your physician. If you experience pain, shortness of breath or dizziness, stop exercising and call a physician.

7 MAIN WORKOUT: AEROBIC&ANAEROBIC

"What you believe and conceive. . . you can achieve."-
Anonymous

B iking, running (do your knees a favor and stay off the pavement!), speed hiking, stair climbers, and "ski specific" machines such as Nordic Track and Nordic Sport are good aerobic exercises. I am going to show you how to make each of these activities "ski specific" so you will get much more than just the aerobic benefit.

SKI SPECIFIC BENEFITS
Shifting weight from ski to ski
Angulation

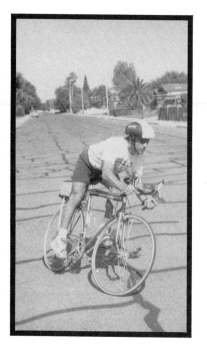

SKI SPECIFIC BIKING

Bike riding is my favorite activity for building aerobic endurance. It is less stressful on knees than running, and the pedalling action is similar to changing weight from foot to foot in skiing. It's also a great means of transportation. So save the environment and ride your bike. . . just make sure you wear a helmet.

To make biking "ski specific", don't ride in a straight line. Instead, make long smooth turns as if you are skiing. Turning a bike is like turning skis, but instead of metal edges gripping the terrain, rubber tires do the job. At the start of each turn, rise off the seat as if you were unweighting skis. Then lean into the turn, driving down on the outside pedal until your turn is completed. There! You just used the same technique on your bike that you do on your skis.

SKI SPECIFIC BENEFITS
Negotiating the Terrain

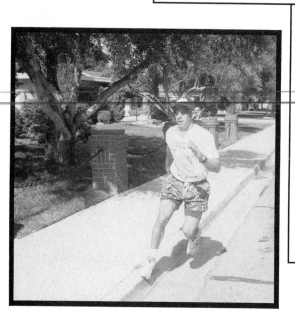

SKI SPECIFIC RUNNING

To make running "ski specific", pretend you are in a slalom course. Imagine where you want to make each turn, then commit to it by pushing hard with your outside foot as you begin the turn and create angles with your body. Instead of a typical stride, run more side-to-side. If you're running on the street push off the side of a curve. This will help train the muscles in a very "ski specific" way. I'm not suggesting you run like this for the entire time. Just add these "ski specific" styles of running in intervals.

SKI SPECIFIC SPEED HIKING

Hiking over a beautiful trail is a great way to spend a day. Besides leaving your stress behind, you get a great workout. To make speed hiking "ski specific", jump on small boulders and walk on fallen trees. This type of speed hiking will increase your balance, agility, and coordination needed for skiing. Make sure you wear hiking boots that give your ankles extra support.

SKI SPECIFIC BENEFITS
Shifting weight from ski to ski
Angulation

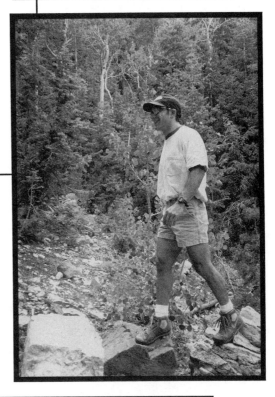

SKI SPECIFIC BENEFITS
Shifting weight from ski to ski
Angulation

SKI SPECIFIC STAIRMASTER

Next time you jump on a stairmaster, don't grab onto the rails for balance. Instead, pretend you are holding poles and concentrate on shifting weight from foot to foot while maintaining balance. This is a tough one, but with a little practice, you will be able to do it with your eyes closed.

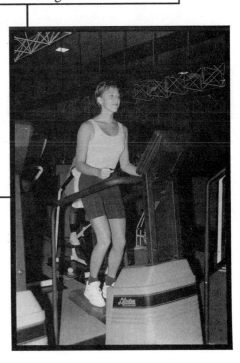

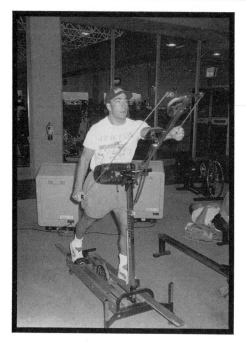

SKI SPECIFIC BENEFITS
Shifting weight from ski to ski
Angulation

NORDIC TRACK

Nordic Track has been around for several years and is highly regarded among skiing and fitness professionals. Along with giving you a great aerobic workout, Nordic Track will help strengthen your legs, arms, stomach, and torso in a very "ski specific" way.

For information call:

(800)328-5888

NORDIC SPORT

will be discussed in the "Home Work Out" chapter.

ANAEROBICS

Aerobics involves low intensity, long duration activity; anaerobics involves high intensity, short duration activity. The best way to train for anaerobic capacity is by *interval* training.

Interval training is holding a steady pace and then increasing to maximum effort for a short time. For example, when you ride your bike, keep a nice steady pace (minimum 80 rpm) on the flats and sprint up hills as fast as you can. Or, when you run, sprint every tenth light pole. Interval training breaks the monotony of any activity and is best for improving your cardiovascular system.

WARNING: Before beginning any exercise program, consult with your physician. If you experience pain, shortness of breath or dizziness, stop exercising and call a physician. Weight training can lead to injury if not done properly. If you are unfamiliar with an exercise seek out a professional trainer to demonstrate the proper technique. A trainer can also help determine safe weight ranges. Always use a "spotter" (someone to help you lift the weight if your muscles fail) when performing the bench press and squat.

8 SKI SPECIFIC WEIGHT TRAINING

" Good timber does not grow with ease: the stronger the wind, the stronger the trees."-J. Willard Marriott

When people think of skiers, they imagine people with big, strong, powerful legs. While strong legs are needed for skiing, overall body strength is also crucial and should not be overlooked. The best way to increase your strength is by training with weights.

For skiing you also need muscle endurance. Endurance is gained by training with light weight and high repetitions (15—30), while strength is achieved with heavy weight and low repetitions (1—8). Both are important for skiing, but you should train for endurance first and strength second.

QUADRICEPS

MUSCLES TRAINED:

Front upper leg and glutemus maximus

LEG PRESS

*in a seated position, press weight in smooth motion by extending and contracting legs

*do not lock knees

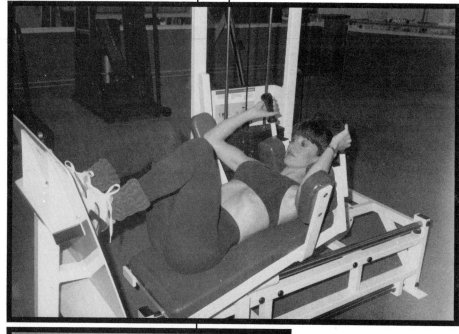

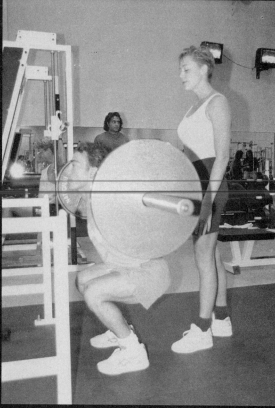

SQUATS

*in a standing position, press shoulder blades together and place bar behind head on lower part of shoulders

*place legs greater than shoulder width apart with toes pointed slightly outwards

*squat keeping head up and back straight, then return to starting position

*do not squat below 90 degrees

SKI SPECIFIC BENEFITS
Raise, lower and
hold ski positions

STEP-UPS

*in a standing position, press shoulder blades together and place bar behind head on lower part of shoulders

*alternating legs, step up onto bench with one leg at a time (height of bench must not allow knee to bend greater than 90 degrees), then return to original position

*do not lock knees

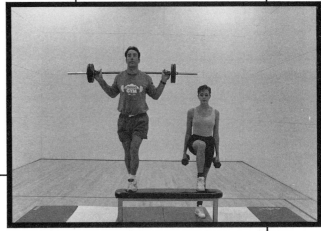

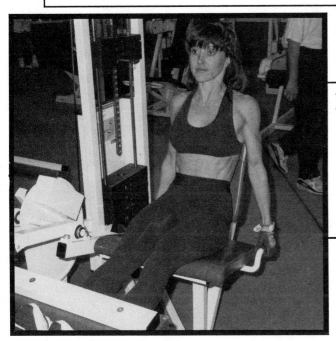

LEG EXTENSIONS

*Adjust machine so pad rests on ankle

*extend legs in smooth motion, then return to original position

*do not lock knees

SINGLE LEG SQUATS

*in a standing position, place one foot on bench (height of bench must not allow knee to bend greater than 90 degrees) and other foot in front of bench

*keeping back straight and head up, bend front knee

*do not bend knee below 90 degrees

*to help keep balanced, focus vision on object in distance

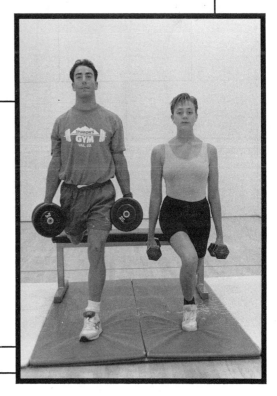

HAMSTRINGS
MUSCLES TRAINED:
Back of upper legs

SKI SPECIFIC BENEFITS:
Raise, lower, and hold ski positions. Improve quickness and balance

LEG CURLS
*adjust pad of machine to touch above heel

*keeping seat down, draw feet to seat

BACK
MUSCLES TRAINED:
Latisimus Dorsi (Lats)

SKI SPECIFIC BENEFITS:
Holding ski positions, maintaining balance

PULL DOWNS
*in a seated position, grip suspended overhead bar wider than shoulder width

*pull down bar in smooth motion

*alternate pulling down bar in front and in back of neck

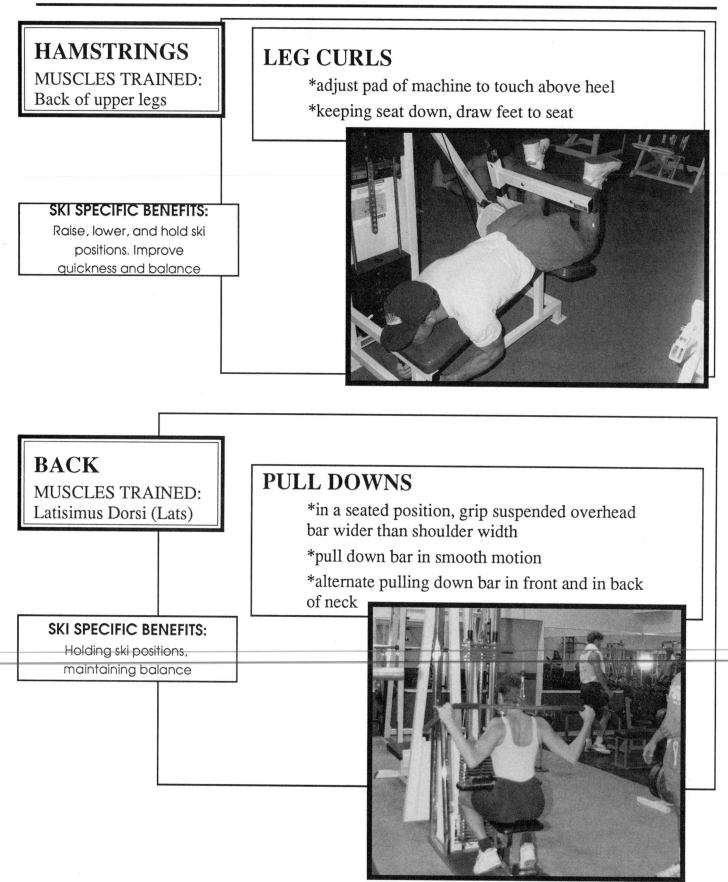

CHEST AND SHOULDERS
MUSCLES TRAINED:
Pectoids and Deltoids

BENCH PRESS

*lying flat on back on bench,
grip bar wider than shoulder width

*keeping feet flat on ground, lower bar
slowly to top of chest

*press weight up and towards rack

*do not lift seat off bench

SKI SPECIFIC BENEFITS:
Pole usage, getting up.
Stabilizing upper body.

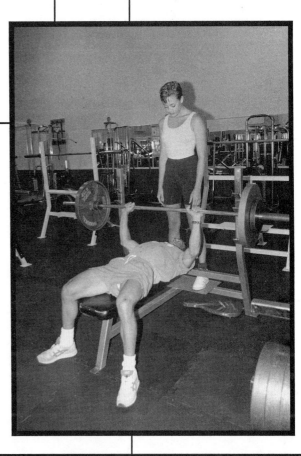

SHOULDER PRESS

*in seated position, grip bar wider
than shoulder width and begin by
placing behind neck on shoulders

*Keeping back straight, press weight
overhead until arms are fully extended

*alternate lowering weight in front
and behind neck

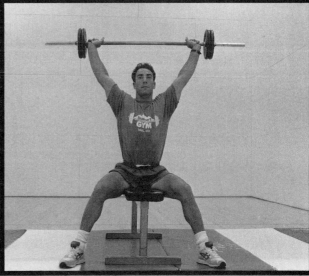

TRICEPS

MUSCLES TRAINED:
Back of upper arms

PUSHDOWNS

*in a standing position, keeping elbows close to body (with lower arms at 90 degrees to body), holding bar with hands, push down on bar

*don't raise bar higher than mid-chest

SKI SPECIFIC BENEFITS:

Pole usage, getting up

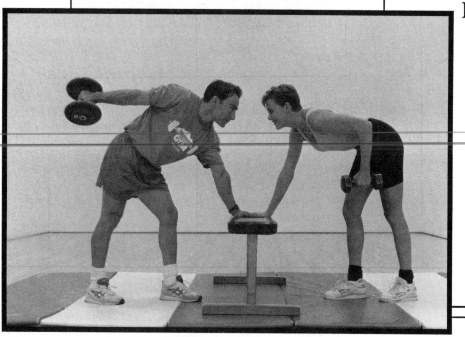

KICKBACKS

*in a standing position, bending forward from waist, support body with one hand on bench

*keeping elbow parallel to ground, raise dumbbell weight until fully extended behind you

SEATED TOE RAISES

*with weight on knees, press down with toes while lifting heels, pausing at top and stretching at bottom

CALVES
MUSCLES TRAINED:
Back of lower legs

SKI SPECIFIC BENEFITS:
Foot control for steering

SHINS
MUSCLES TRAINED:
Front of lower leg

SKI SPECIFIC BENEFITS:
Initiate turns, steer skis, stabilization, edge control, lifting ski tips

NOTE:
Lower leg is extremely important to skiing

FLEX WALK

*in a standing position, flex feet so only heel is on ground

*walk with straight legs

(it is more difficult going down hill)

STOMACH

all stomach exercises should be done on a soft surface (mats, rubber weight lifting floors, gymnastics floors, and grass are all good).

MUSCLES TRAINED:

Abdominals

CRUNCHES

*lying on back, bend knees and place lower legs on bench

*cross arms over chest and raise upper body

*lower upper body not allowing shoulders to touch ground

PHOTOS THIS PAGE

RIGHT:
Starting Position

LEFT:
Finishing Position

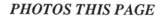

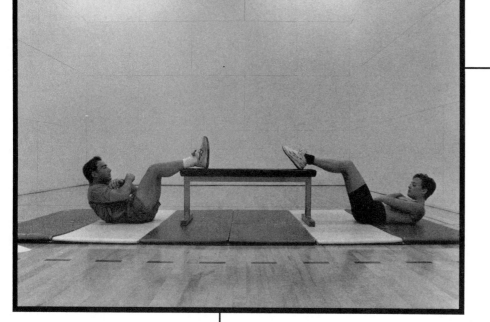

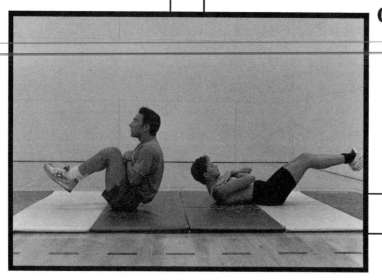

CLAM-UPS

*lay on back with feet and shoulders off ground and knees bent

*cross arms over chest and raise upper body and knees simultaneously to meet

V-UPS

*lay on back with feet and shoulders off ground and knees slightly bent

*with arms straight back and covering ears, raise upper and lower body simultaneously touching hands to toes

TOP PHOTO THIS PAGE

RIGHT:
Starting Position

LEFT:
Finishing Position

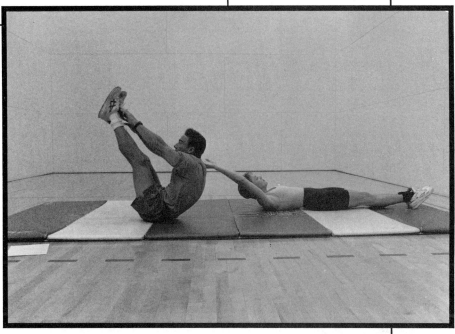

BIKERS

*laying on back, place hands behind head with legs raised and knees slightly bent

*raise upper and lower body simultaneously touching elbow to opposite knee alternating sides

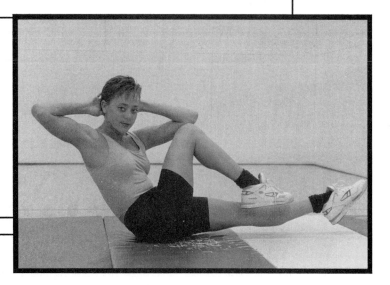

ABDUCTORS AND ADDUCTORS

MUSCLES TRAINED:
Hip angulators

SKI SPECIFIC BENEFITS:
Edging and angulation

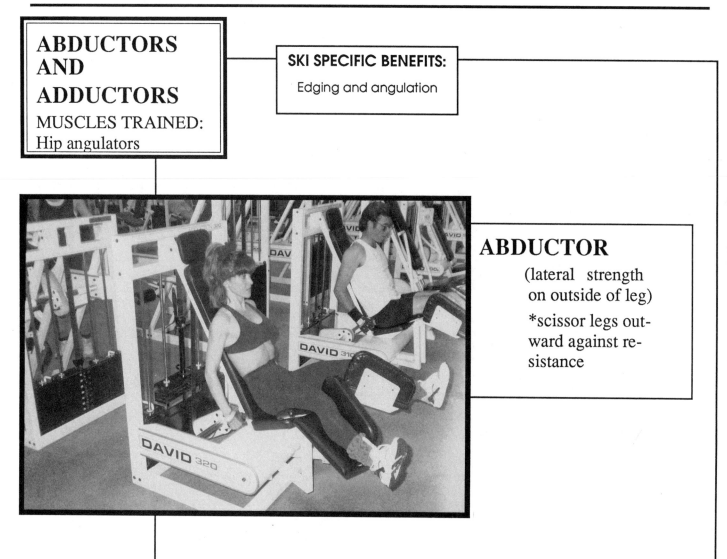

ABDUCTOR

(lateral strength on outside of leg)

*scissor legs outward against resistance

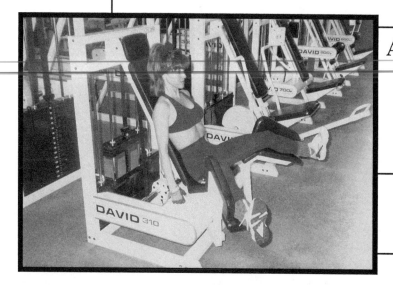

ADDUCTOR

(lateral strength on inside of leg)

*scissor legs inward against resistance

Power training is the most fun, it is an advanced form of exercises. Before you begin, you should have a high level of aerobic/anaerobic,.strength, and strength endurance. Proceed with caution as power training places a lot of stress on your body. Only perform these exercises on a soft surface (mats, rubber weight lifting floors, gymnastics floors, and grass are all good).

9 SKI SPECIFIC POWER TRAINING

"Everything that enlarges the sphere of human powers, that shows man he can do what he thought he could not do, is valuable."—Ben Johnson

Once you become an intermediate level skier, the sport requires explosive reactive movements that necessitate quick changes in direction from up to down or side to side. You need strong muscles, but they must be quick as well (think of skiing a bump run).

While strength training involves moving a mass a distance with no consideration to time, power training incorporates both strength and speed (or quickness). The element of time becomes a very important factor. Exercises that train your body in quick, explosive, powerful movements are called *plyometrics*. They are high level forms of bouncing and skipping.

For the past two years, I have taught a SKI SHAPE class at a local health club. Plyometrics are the overwhelming favorite part of my class with my students. Along with increasing your power and quickness, these drills also improve coordination, balance, and agility by leaps and bounds. . . literally!

With all plyometric exercises it is important to keep your stomach muscles tight and your focus straight ahead. While performing these exercises try to avoid extra movements with your body (just as if you were skiing).

GLUTS AND LEGS

MUSCLES TRAINED:
Upper and lower legs.

SQUAT JUMPS

*start in standing position with knees bent 90 degrees and hands held in front (like you're holding ski polls)

*spring upward making slow and controlled landings but never coming to a full stop or letting your knees bend past 90 degrees

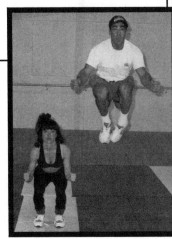

TOP:
Absorb landing impact with your toes

BOTTOM:
Be sure your feet clear the bench

SKI SPECIFIC BENEFITS:

Explosive power to drive through turns. Retraction, extension for bumps. Overall agility for advanced skiing

BENCH JUMPS

(At first this is a tough one; but stick with it. After a few weeks, you'll be well on your way to becoming a mogul monster.)

*start in standing position with knees slightly bent and hands held in front (like you're holding ski polls) about two feet away from a bench of a height you can comfortably jump over

*while jumping over the bench keep hands in same position lifting knees as close to chest as possible, then extend legs towards ground to land

*without stopping rebound back and forth off of toes rather than absorbing landings in a flat-footed position

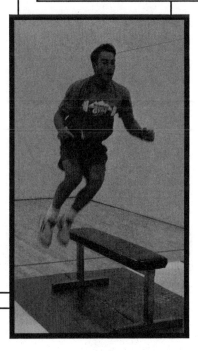

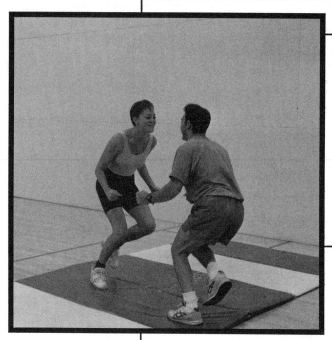

LATERAL JUMPS

*starting in standing position with knees slightly bent and hands held in front (like you're holding ski polls), jump laterally from one leg to the other as quickly as possible

(to increase challenge, touch your hand on floor next to foot)

TOP:
Push off with outside foot while inclining body towards other side

BOTTOM:
Left figure is in starting position, right figure is preparing to switch legs

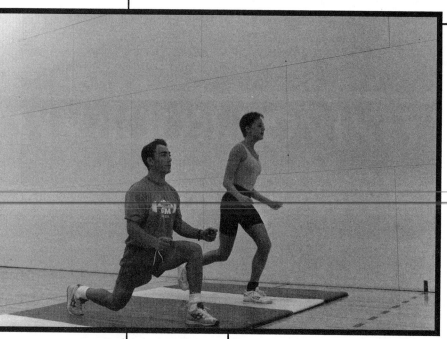

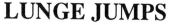

LUNGE JUMPS

*in lunge position, extend hands out in front (like holding ski polls)

*jump up and out, switching legs in air, landing softly in starting position

(don't let front knee bend below 90 degrees)

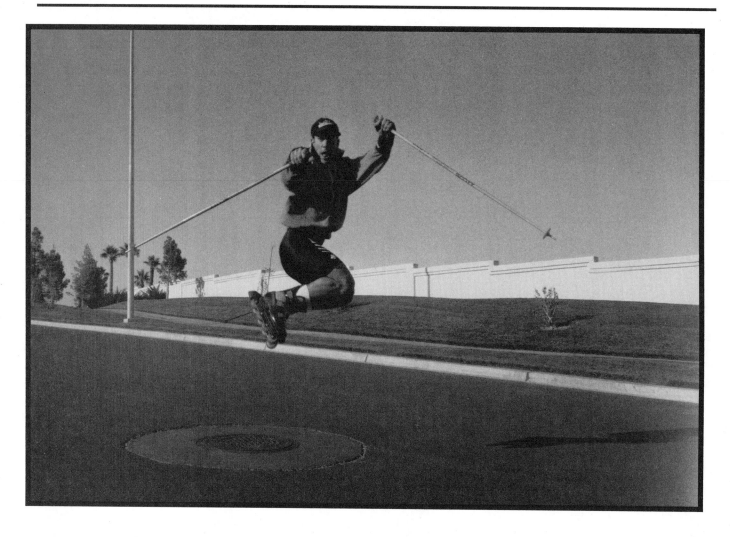

10 SKI SPECIFIC CROSS TRAINING

"Man is not the sum of what he has but the totality of what he does not yet have, of what he might have."—Jean Paul Sartre

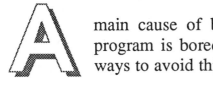main cause of burnout in a training program is boredom. One of the best ways to avoid this is by cross training.

What is cross training? It's a 'sexy' term brilliant marketers coined to describe an age-old practice, participating in one sport to help you improve in another. They coined it to sell more shoes and give us all an excuse to buy fashionable workout clothes we don't need. With this in mind, let's look at some sports that *will* help your skiing in very specific ways. The main cross training sports useful for skiing are in-line-skating (commonly referred to as rollerblading), mountain biking, and mountain running.

IN-LINE-SKATING

I tried on my first pair of Rollerblade skates two years ago and was immediately hooked! I can't think of any other activity that simulates downhill skiing as well as in-line-skating. When you practice ski turns with them, you are exercising the same muscles used in skiing, in the same fashion, and having just as much fun. What more can you ask for?! The skating action alone is one of the best exercises to promote independent leg action vital for good skiing.

In-line skating is such good preparation for skiing that 150 members of the U.S. Ski Team currently use Rollerblade skates as a fun supplement to their dryland training On a health note, skating puts very little stress on your body while providing a great "ski specific" workout.

Along with "ski specific" conditioning, it's an opportunity to refine technique. The polyurethane wheels hold like a perfectly edged ski. Skating down a well paved road is like skiing down a groomed hill on fresh tuned skis

Rollerblade has just developed a new skate called the Slolomblade. It is the first skate designed specifically for skate-ski use. It has five wheels for greater speed and a full boot (very similar to your ski boot) for lateral stability.

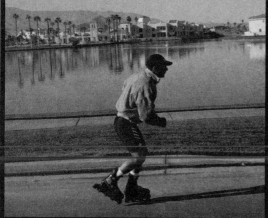

To start find smooth flat terrain (an empty parking lot is ideal) and practice basic skating technique. Once you get rolling, you will eventually need to stop. All skates come with rear brake. After you become a more skilled skater, you will find other ways to stop.

Once you learn the basic skating technique and are able to make parallel (or close to it) turns on skis, you can 'skate-ski'. You don't need a very steep hill. A smooth road with a 5-15 degree pitch will get the adrenalin rushing. The best way to achieve "ski specific" training is to practice 'skate-skiing' downhill and do all out sprints going up. This is a form of interval training and will greatly improve your anaerobic shape.

MOUNTAIN BIKING

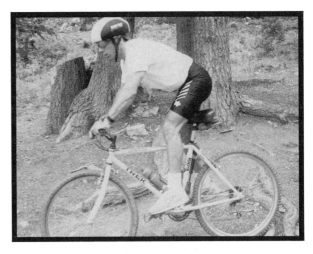

Mountain biking is another great way to get in SKI SHAPE. It demands balance, coordination, concentration, and the ability to read the terrain like you do in skiing. Make your rides more fun by coasting downhill, keeping a nice even pace (80 rpm) on the flats, and sprinting uphill.

MOUNTAIN RUNNING

Mountain running is different than your average jog around the park. Mountain running focuses on agil-

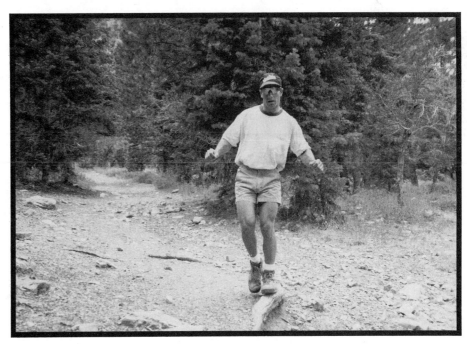

ity and quickness as well as providing an aerobic/ anaerobic workout. And, like when skiing, you will have to adjust to the changes in the terrain in order to stay in balance.

I hate street running. It's about as

boring as watching bad re-runs of THE DAVID LET-TERMAN SHOW. However, throw in some trees, rocks, streams, and other obstacles and give the terrain some vertical drops and rises. . . now that's fun!

The key to good "ski specific" mountain running is using your imagination. Run around trees like you are skiing a slalom course. Jump from rock to rock as if skiing bumps, and run across fallen logs like skiing a narrow chute.

Other cross-training sports great for skiing are:

*Trampoline—for body awareness and control

*Tennis—for footwork and lateral agility

*Sand volleyball—quickness and power(not to mention a great tan)

*Soccer—sharp efficient movements (changes of direction)

*Windsurfing— great for balance

WARNING: Before beginning any exercise program, consult with your physician. If you experience pain, shortness of breath or dizziness, stop exercising and call a physician.

11 TRAINING PROGRAM

" The great end of life is not knowledge but action."-
Thomas Henry Huxley

et's be realistic. Most of us simply don't have time to train five or six days a week. Does this mean you shouldn't train at all? Absolutely not!

Anything is better than nothing as long as you use good judgement and common sense. I would suspect that eighty percent of you should start out with the green program while the other twenty percent may be ready for the blue or black. Whichever program you choose, keep in mind that you don't do every type of training each work out. I have given you a guideline to follow with different exercises from different categories. You may choose to do cardiovascular one day and weights another or combine both on some days. The important thing is to plug in the different forms of exercises in the way that works for you best. Above all things. . . keep your conditioning goals realistic.

BEGINNER PROGRAM (GREEN)

Train 2 days/week 1 hour/day. Rest 2 days in between work-outs

<u>Weeks</u>: 1-2— Aerobics both days, weights 1 day

3-8— Aerobics 1 day, anaerobics 1 day, weights 2 days

9-12— Aerobics/anaerobics, weights (endurance 1 day strength 1 day), cross training

INTERMEDIATE PROGRAM (BLUE)

Train 3 days/week

<u>Weeks</u>: 1-2— Aerobics 2 days/week, weights (endurance) 2 days/week, cross train 1 day/week

3-5— Aerobics/anaerobics 2 days/week, weights (endurance) 3 days/week, cross train 1 day/week

6-12— Aerobics/anaerobics 2 or 3 days/week, weights (2 days endurance 1 day strength), cross train 2 days/week

ADVANCED PROGRAM (BLACK)

Train 5 days/week

<u>Weeks</u>: 1-12—Aerobics/anaerobics, weights, power training, cross training

BEGINNER (Green)

ACTIVITY	EXERCISE	MIN/REPS	NOTES
Warm-Up	Jumping Jacks Jump Rope Running in place	5min	do only 1 warm-up exercise per day
Stretch	Pike Stradle Knee Bender Pelican Sumo chicken Wing Single Knee Wall Hold Tuck Far Reach Four Points	5min	do only 1 stretch per body part
Aerobics/Anaerobics	Speed Hiking Stair Master Biking	20min	do only 1 exercise per day
Weight Training	**(UPPER BODY)** Bench Press Tricep Pushdown Shoulder Press Pull Down **(LOWER BODY)** Leg Extension Leg Press Leg Curl Seated Toe Raise Flex Walk **(STOMACH)** Crunch	(Endurance) 3sets-12 to 15reps (Strength) 3sets-2 to 5reps (For stomach do 3sets-25reps)	do only 2 exercises for Upper Body and 2 for Lower Body/day
Cross Training	In-Line Skating Mountain Biking Mountain Running KneedSpeed Sand Volleyball Tennis Trampoline	30min	skate, bike, and run on easy terrain *skate, bike, run, and KneedSpeed can always be substituted for Aerobic / Anaerobic exercises
Cool Down	Stretch	5min	don't forget to cool down. . .it's important!

ADVANCED WORKOUT (BLACK DIAMOND) ➡️

INTERMEDIATE WORKOUT (BLUE) ▼

ACTIVITY	EXERCISE	MIN/REPS	NOTES
Warm-Up	Jumping Jacks Jump Rope Running in place	5min	do only 1 warm-up exercise per day
Stretch	Pike Stradle Knee Bender Pelican Sumo chicken Wing Single Knee Wall Hold Tuck Far Reach Four Points	5min	do only 1 stretch per body part
Aerobics/Anaerobics	Speed Hiking Stair Master Biking Nordic Track	20min	do only 1 exercise per day
Weight Training	**(UPPER BODY)** Bench Press Tricep Pushdown Tricep Kickback Shoulder Press Pull Down **(LOWER BODY)** Leg Extension Leg Press Leg Curl Seated Toe Raise Flex Walk Single Leg Squat Abductor Adductor **(STOMACH)** Crunch Clam-up	(Endurance) 3sets-12 to 15reps (Strength) 3sets-2 to 5reps (For stomach do 3sets-35reps)	do only 3 exercises for Upper Body and 3 for Lower Body/day
Cross Training	In-Line Skating Mountain Biking Mountain Running KneedSpeed Sand Volleyball Tennis Trampoline	30min	skate, bike, and run on intermediate terrain *skate, bike, run, and Kneed-Speed can always be substituted for Aerobic/Anaerobic exercises As soon as you feel comfortable, use poles and skate ski
Cool Down	Stretch	5min	don't forget to cool down. . .it's important!

ACTIVITY	EXERCISE	MIN/REPS	NOTES
Warm-Up	Jumping Jacks Jump Rope Running in place	5min	do only 1 warm-up exercise per day
Stretch	Pike Stradle Knee Bender Pelican Sumo chicken Wing Single Knee Wall Hold Tuck Far Reach Four Points	5min	do more dynamic and partner stretching
Aerobics/Anaerobics	Speed Hiking Stair Master Biking Nordic Track	30-45min	do only 1 exercise per day
Weight Training	**(UPPER BODY)** Bench Press Tricep Pushdown Tricep Kickback Shoulder Press Pull Down **(LOWER BODY)** Squat Step-Up Leg Extension Leg Press Leg Curl Seated Toe Raise Flex Walk Single Leg Squat Abductor Adductor **(STOMACH)** Crunch Clam-Up V-Up Bicycle	(Endurance) 4sets-12 to 15reps (Strength) 4sets-2 to 5reps (For stomach do 4sets-50reps)	don't train upper and lower body in the same day
Power Training	Squat Jump Bench Jump Lateral Jump Lunge Jump	3-5sets-10-12reps	this type of training is more advanced and strenuous to the body; minimum two days rest between power training sessions
Cross Training	In-Line Skating Mountain Biking Mountain Running KneedSpeed Sand Volleyball Tennis Trampoline	30min-1 hr	skate, bike, and run on difficult terrain *skate, bike, run, and Kneed-Speed can always be sub-stituted for Aerobic/Anaerobic exercises As soon as you feel comfort-able, use poles and skate ski
Cool Down	Stretch	5min	don't forget to cool down. . .it's important!

WARNING: Before beginning any exercise program, consult with your physician. If you experience pain, shortness of breath or dizziness, stop exercising and call a physician.

12 ON SNOW WARM UP

"There are two things to aim at in life: first, to get what you want; and, after that, to enjoy it."—Logan Pearsall Smith

Although competitive skiers spend up to an hour warming up before their event, most recreational skiers avoid warming up like the plague. They will spend hours in the car or plane, unload their equipment, and jump right into the lift line. Just like warming up before a workout, it is even more important to warm-up before skiing! Warming up will give you the readiness feeling that will help both physically and psychologically. Following are some warm-up and stretching exercises you can do 'on snow' before your first run or any time your muscles get cold (i.e. after a long break or lunch).

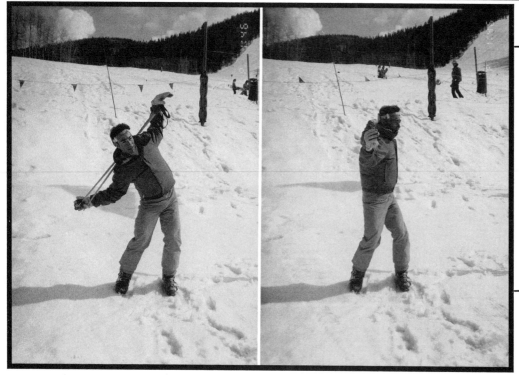

TRUNK TWIST

*placing ski polls behind neck, stand with legs about shoulder width apart

*twist trunk and bend side-to-side,

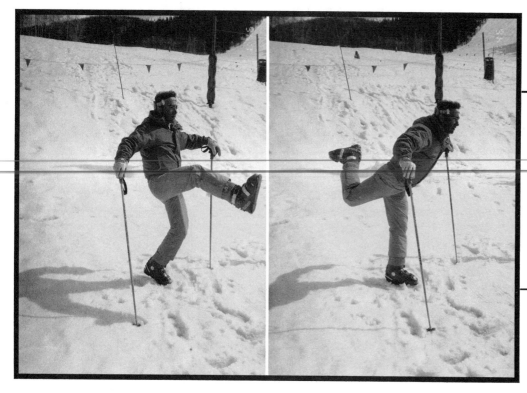

LEG KICKS

*in a standing position, using ski polls for balance, kick leg forward and back (repeat with other leg)

ARM CIRCLES

   *vigorously swing arms in large circles

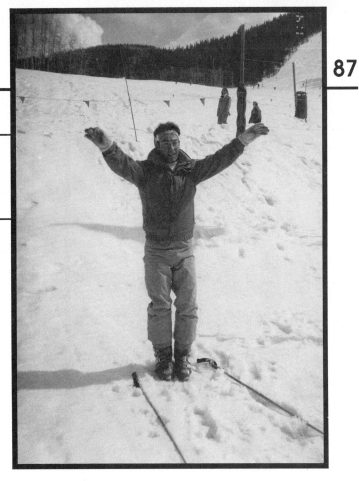

SIDE LUNGE

   *standing with skis shoulder width apart, keep one leg straight and bend knee of other leg to the side (repeat with other leg)

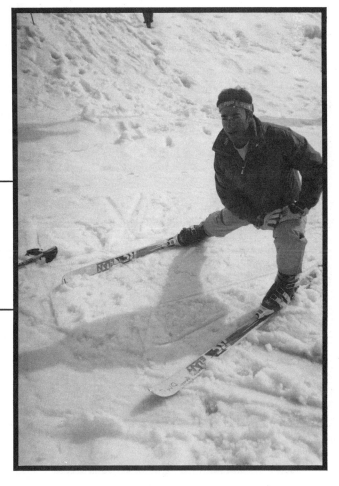

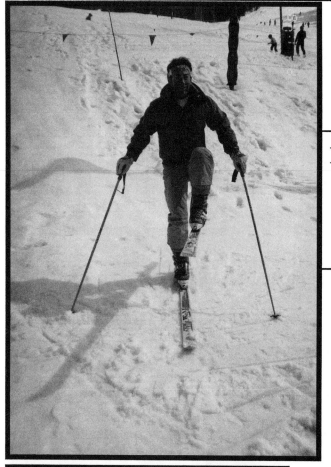

KNEE LIFT

   *standing with skis about 6 inches apart, plant poles by outside of boots

   *keeping back straight, lift knee toward chest as far as possible

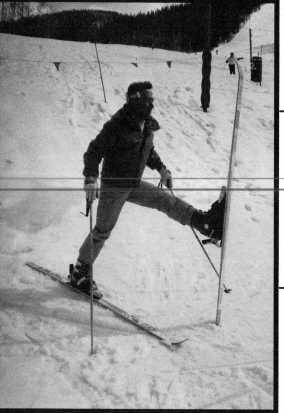

HAMSTRING STRETCH

   *using poles for balance, lift one ski in front so the tail rests in the snow and the tip is pointing straight up

   *keeping your back straight, push your pelvic area forward until you feel a stretch in your hamstring

---

WARNING: Before beginning any exercise program, consult with your physician. If you experience pain, shortness of breath or dizziness, stop exercising and call a physician.

13 HOME WORK OUT

"Do what you can, with what you have, where you are." -Theodore Roosevelt

Having a gym to work out in is great, but if you don't belong to one you can still get in great SKI SHAPE.

I know what you're thinking. . . more push-ups and sit-ups. Actually those are good exercises and should be part of any fitness routine, but the home work out I'm about to show you goes beyond these few basic exercises.

All.you need is a Sport Cord, Kneedspeed, and a new machine from the makers of NordicTrack called The NordicSport Downhill. These three things and a few other ski-specific exercises that I will show you will get you in the best SKI SHAPE of your life!.

Even if you do go to a gym, you might want to incorporate the home work out into your routine. It's a great way to vary your training and keep things from getting dull.

SPORT CORD

The Sport Cord is a piece of latex surgical tubing with special attachments which let you perform a variety of "ski specific" exercises. (Sport Cord is a registered trademark of Sport Cord Inc. of Vail, CO) The following exercises have been developed by one of the most respected ski training teams in the U.S. and are used by some of the top racers on the World Cup Circuit. The team that developed the exercises consists of:

DR. RICHARD STEADMAN Internationally recognized orthopedic surgeon and Chairman and Chief Physician of the U.S. Ski Team

TOPPER HAGERMAN, Ph.D. Trainer of the successful U.S. Men's Alpine Ski Team from 1982 to 1984. Now a sports medicine consultant in Vail, CO.

JOHN ATKINS Director of the U.S. Ski Team from 1988 to 1991. Now works as a sports medicine consultant in Vail, CO with Topper Hagerman.

The Sport Cord is very easy to use and comes complete with handles, foot straps, belt, and door attachment. Before you begin your ski specific training, know your fitness level. If you're not sure what your fitness level is, **consult with your physician.**

THE SPORT CORD EXERCISES

There are about 11 ski-specific Sport Cord exercises. All of them are excellent but the following two are the ones that I think you will get the most out of. With all the Sport Cord exercises, try to maintain good ski form: look straight ahead, keep your knees slightly bent, and your back straight.

If your goal is to build muscle, use additional resistance. If you're trying to tone your muscles, do more repetitions with less resistance. Remember, always warm up and stretch before your Sport Cord work out and cool down and stretch afterwards.

Ski Dip

*place outside foot on cord 12 to 20 inches from handle

*slightly bend knee and pull handle to waist

*raise other foot off floor and place two fingers on back of chair (use chair for balance only)

*Slowly lower to a 1/3 knee bend

*return to starting position (always keep slight bend in working leg)

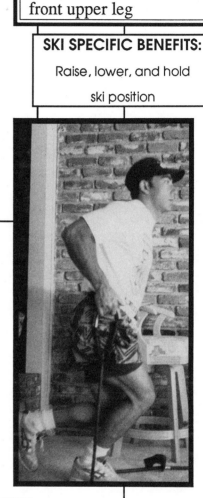

MUSCLES TRAINED:
front upper leg

SKI SPECIFIC BENEFITS:
Raise, lower, and hold ski position

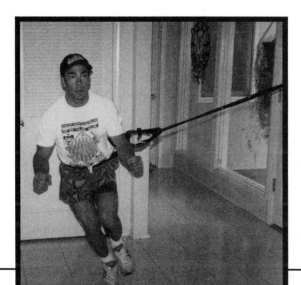

Ski Step

*attach Sport Cord at medium height in door jamb

*run belt through both handles and fasten belt around waist

*step 6 to 7 feet away from door

*assume a low angulated "ski" position with side to door (simulate poling motion with arms)

*begin with foot closest to door and jump to other foot

*pause and jump back to starting position

MUSCLES TRAINED
upper and lower leg

SKI SPECIFIC BENEFITS:
Maintain ski position, turn and jump

Kneedspeed

This is a really fun exercise to do. The Kneedspeed is basically a 6 foot long by 2 feet wide sliding surface. It can be rolled up and stored away and is perfect for training your muscles in a ski-specific way. Again, there are many exercises you can do on the Kneedspeed but the following is the best overall work-out.

Kneedspeed Slide Exercise

*place booties over shoes. Flat sole athletic shoes work best

*Stand on the Kneedspeed with both feet together and the outside foot touching the block.

*bend knees and simultaneously step toward the opposite block and push off block your foot is presently against. Remember to push off with your entire leg, all the way up to your hip. Do not push with just your ankle.

*be sure to keep your feet apart while sliding. The proper position is to have your feet wider than shoulder width. Do not bring your feet together until your lead foot has hit the opposite block

*start slowly at first until you are comfortable with the motion. The exercise is designed to be done at an 18-22 rpm. Any faster and you will become anaerobic.

For more information call Kneedspeed at 1-800-523-7674

MUSCLES TRAINED:
Inner thigh and hip

SKI SPECIFIC BENEFITS

Angulation, rotary push off balance, agility, and cardiovascular

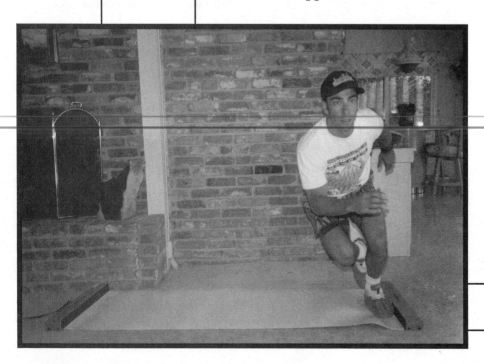

NordicSport

The NordicSport is from the same people who make NordicTrack. It is designed to educate your body to make the right skiing moves. This "ski specific" trainer provides off-snow training to enhance your skiing skills through improved body awareness, and physical conditioning. It can be used by skiers of any level, regardless of whether they're first learning and need light resistance at a low decline (bunny hill) or heavy resistance at a steep decline (black diamond).

NordicSport Downhill Exercise

*adjust tension and elevation settings to the lightest and lowest grade

*step onto the device on the supportive step and place one foot into footplate. Then place the other.

*grasp pole handles in a position where the arms are spread in front slightly wider than your body. As you pivot your heels to the right, your right hand should thrust forward to "plant the pole". At the same time draw your left hand-grip back slightly.

*your forward lean should be such that your torso is perpendicular to the incline on the simulator.

*NOTE: The NordicSport comes complete with a video tape and manual.

MUSCLES TRAINED:
All major muscle groups

SKI SPECIFIC BENEFITS:

Steering, edging, pressure, balance, agility

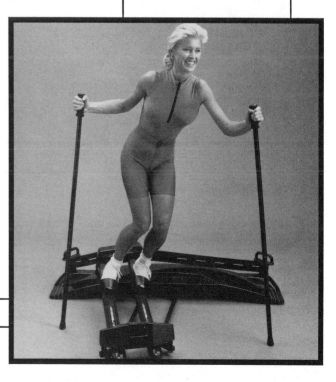

MUSCLES TRAINED:
Front of lower leg, ankle

SKI SPECIFIC BENEFITS:

Steering

Lower Leg Strengthener

*in a seated position with legs straight, place the inside of your foot against a solid object.

*using your hands for support, use your foot and lower leg to push against object (foot should be at a slight angle).

*hold for thirty seconds and switch legs.

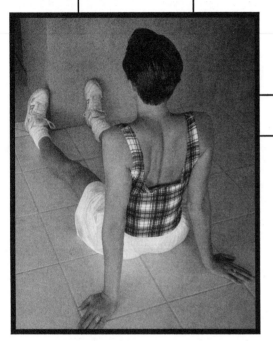

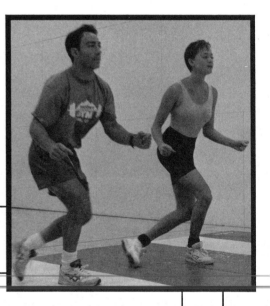

MUSCLES TRAINED:
Gluts, upper and lower legs

SKI SPECIFIC BENEFITS:

Quick turns and adjustments

Cross Overs

*in a standing position, bend knees slightly and hold arms like you hold ski poles.

*step sideways by crossing feet front to back.

*keep working at this until you can take several steps in each direction at a quick pace (this will really help your agility)

Chair Dips

*set up three chairs in a triangle shape

*supporting your weight on the arms of two chairs, put your feet on the third

*keeping your stomach and seat tight, bend your elbows (try to hit 90 degrees) and push back up

MUSCLES TRAINED: Back of upper arms (triceps), shoulders, trunk region

SKI SPECIFIC BENEFITS: Pole usage, turn initiation

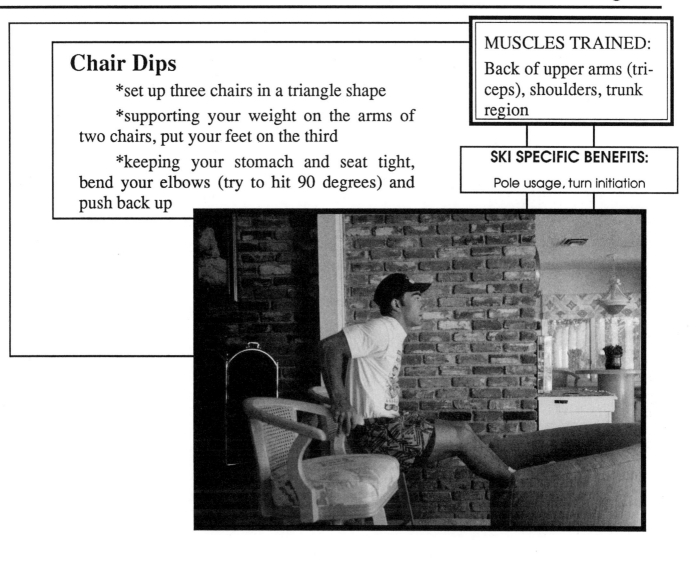

If you do these exercises correctly and stick to a consistent program, working out at home can drastically improve your SKI SHAPE! Along with these "ski specific" home exercises, all the exercises in the "Power Training" chapter can be done at home. Just remember, plyometrics are an advanced form of exercise and caution should be taken.

Even if you like to work out in a gym with weights, you may want to try a few home work outs. Remember, the more options and creativity you have in training, the less likely you will burn out.

14

SKIING SKILLS

"As I understand it, sport is hard work for which you do not get paid."—Irvin S. Cobb

In the chapter titled "Analysis of a Skiers Needs", I talked briefly about the major physiological components of skiing. In this chapter, I am going to explain the basic skills needed in all levels of skiing, whether you're a beginner or on the World Cup Circuit, as they apply to those components.

This isn't confusing, although it certainly sounds that way. After reading these next few pages, you will have a much better understanding of the skills used in skiing. And of the exercises in this book you may want to concentrate on!

The main skills in skiing are balance, rhythm, flow, rotary, edging, and pressure control

BALANCE

Balance is the ability to maintain equilibrium as your body changes position.

If you have difficulty with balance, you may want to concentrate on mountain biking, walking on fallen trees, and in-line skating.

RHYTHM

Rhythm is the ability to appropriately time your turns. If you have ever had an easy time following another skier turn for turn, they probably had good rhythm. The best way to improve your rhythm is to skate/ski. Put on some music and make turns to the beat of the music. The faster the music, the quicker the turns. Another good exercise is lateral jumps varying your rhythm from set to set.

FLOW

Flow is how you move your body from turn to turn. Do you get stuck on the backs of your skis or does your body move into the new turn? Try "ski specific" biking if your flow needs improvement.

ROTARY

Rotary is steering with your feet. Many people try to turn with every part of their body except their feet. To improve your rotary skills, work on flex walks and lower leg strengtheners.

EDGING

Edging happens when you turn your ski on its side. It is also the only way you can make a clean carved turn as opposed to keeping your skis flat and doing a controlled skid. In-line skating is a great way to hone your edging.

PRESSURE CONTROL

As you edge your ski, you apply pressure to it. This bends the ski and gives your turn shape. The stronger you are, the more pressure you will be able to exert. Step-ups and squats will help you with this.

FINALLY

I only mentioned a few of the "ski specific" exercises that will help you with each skill. If you go back through the exercises and look at the boxes labeled Ski Specific Benefit(s), you should see which exercises may be best for your personal skill level to put you in SKI SHAPE.

WARNING: If you are under a doctor's care, have special health problems or any special dietary needs, please consult your physician before changing what or how you eat.

15 ENERGY FOODS FOR SKIING

"Another good reducing exercise consists in placing both hands against the table edge and pushing back."—Robert Quillen

No matter how hard you train, you won't be able to use your finely tuned muscles unless they are properly fueled. A proper diet is one of the most overlooked aspects of sports performance and yet is absolutely vital! The sad truth is that people put better fuel in their cars than they do in their bodies. Your diet should consist primarily of complex and simple carbohydrates and protein. Limit your fat intake to a minimum and drink at least eight glasses of water a day. Following is a brief overview of the four basic food groups and suggestions for breakfast, lunch, dinner, and snacks.

FOUR BASIC FOOD GROUPS

I. Milk Group—examples of this food group include milk, yogurt, cheese, ice cream

II. Meat Group—examples of this food group include beef, poultry, fish, eggs—limit intake of red meat

III. Vegetable and Fruit Group—examples of this food group include grapefruit, melon, apple, orange, broccoli, spinach, corn

IV. Bread and Cereal Group—examples of this food group include oatmeal, pasta, rice, whole grain bread, dry cereal

BREAKFAST

This is the most important meal of the day. The worst thing you can do is skip breakfast. Eating breakfast helps get your body ready for the activities of the day. Unfortunately many ski areas serve heavy, energy sapping breakfasts such as fried eggs, bacon, ham, and other fatty foods. Keep your ski breakfast low in fat, moderate in protein, and high in carbohydrates. Try a hot bowl of oatmeal topped with fresh fruit, whole wheat pancakes with little or no butter, or poached eggs with whole wheat toast. (There are many healthier substitutes for butter and syrups). To get some vitamin C, wash the meal down with a tall glass of orange juice. These foods are easily digested and will give you instant energy for skiing.

LUNCH

Many of my clients blow it here. They ski with great energy in the morning, then barely make it through the afternoon. Most people accept this. Granted, if you are not in good shape, you may be worn out by afternoon (what a waste, the ski day is just beginning) but you can get a second wind from a good nutritious lunch. It's not a good idea to skip lunch or eat a heavy, high fat lunch that makes you fall asleep on your plate (I've actually seen this happen— but I woke up after a few minutes). Instead, eat a lunch high in carbohydrates such as a baked potato or pasta, and then get some potassium from a banana.

DINNER

Dinner should consist of complex carbohydrates and protein. Try some chicken over brown rice. Or substitute beans, pasta, or fish. Also, keep the alcohol to a minimum. The altitude causes dehydration and alcohol will add to it.

SKI SNACKS

You burn a lot of calories skiing and it's not a bad idea to snack between meals. Your best bets are raisins, bananas, apples, oranges, or all natural granola bars. A Snickers bar here and there won't hurt either.

FLUIDS

Another key to skiing strong all day is drinking plenty of water. If you feel thirsty—it's too late, you are probably already dehydrated. It's a good idea to stop for a water break every few runs. Also, keep the alcohol to a minimum. The altitude causes dehydration and alcohol will add to it. Besides it's not fun skiing with the bottle flu.

OTHER SUGGESTIONS

*Chew food thoroughly to help digest and absorb nutrients

*Avoid foods high in processed sugars (i.e. candy bars). In the long run these will drain energy

*Don't eat meals less than one hour before heavy exercise

*Avoid late night snacks; these can disrupt the sleeping process

*Pay attention to how food is prepared...deep frying adds more fat than steaming or broiling. And avoid heavy sauces and gravies.

16 ASSESSING SKIING LEVEL

"They can because they think they can."—Virgil

I bet the last time someone asked you how good a skier you were, you answered in one of three ways:

Beginner

Intermediate

Advanced

For the most part, these categories are pretty ambiguous. When do you move from beginner to intermediate and from intermediate to advanced or expert? Unfortunately, there are lots of skiers who correlate speed with skill. Many people categorize themselves as advanced, but when you see them ski, they're a beginner turning at MACH 5 speed.

LEVEL SYSTEM 1 THROUGH 9

This level system was designed by the ski teaching industry to assess skiing ability. Only a small number of skiers take lessons, so many never hear of the level system

There are 9 levels. Levels 1 through 3 are beginner; levels 4 through 6 are intermediate; levels 7 through 9 are advanced. Each level includes skills you should be comfortable with before moving on to the next level. Following is a list of the skills you should achieve at each of the 9 levels:

LEVEL 1

Usually your first day on skis. You should be able to walk (with your skis on), stop by using a large wedge (the old term is snow plow), climb, and turn.

LEVEL 2

You should be able to make linked round wedge turns and be able to turn to a complete stop.

LEVEL 3

You should be able to ski in a smaller wedge and use the shape of your turn to controle your speed. You should also start to bring your skis closer together (match) at the end of your turn.

LEVEL 4

You should be able to match your skis earlier in the turn and feel comfortable with the increased speed. You should start to ski easy blue terrain.

LEVEL 5

You should be able to match your skis parallel before you turn across the hill (before the fall line). You should also be able to use different turn shapes and speeds according to the terrain.

LEVEL 6

You should be working on an open parallel turn with a pole plant. You should be comfortable with most blue runs.

LEVEL 7

You should be able to make short radius parallel turns in the fall line, and medium and long radius carved turns across the fall line. You should feel comfortable on groomed single black diamond runs.

LEVEL 8

You should be able to make dynamic parallel turns in all types of snow conditions and terrain including powder and large moguls.

LEVEL 9

You should be able to ski all single diamond and double black diamond runs in all snow conditions and terrain.

17 FINDING A TRAINER

"It's a funny thing about life; if you refuse to accept any-thing but the best, you very often get it."—W. Somerset Maugham

Having a good personal trainer is great! They can really help you stay on the right track A good trainer will tailor specific programs for your goals and make certain you are doing the exercises safely and correctly. Perhaps the biggest benefit of a personal trainer is that they can keep you motivated.

FOUR KEY POINTS

1. be certain they are professionally certified

2. ask for references

3. watch them train their clients to see if you like their style

4. if they don't ask what *your* personal goals are, don't use them

The best way to find a Personal Trainer is to go to a few health clubs near you and ask the front desk. Personal Trainers charge between $25 and $55 an hour, varying with geographic location, reputation, and level of experience and education—and, if they're good, it's money well spent.

BEGINNER (Green)

ACTIVITY	EXERCISE	MIN/REPS	NOTES
Warm-Up			
Stretch			
Aerobics/Anaerobics			
Weight Training			
Cross Training			
Cool Down			

18 YOUR PERSONAL TRAINING CHARTS

"The thing is to be able to outlast the trends."—Paul Anka

Photocopy the charts in this section and use them to keep a record of your actual workout. You can use them along with the charts on pages 80 through 82 to personalize your workout. Have fun!

ADVANCED WORKOUT (BLACK DIAMOND) ➔

INTERMEDIATE WORKOUT (BLUE) ▼

ACTIVITY	EXERCISE	MIN/REPS	NOTES
Warm-Up			
Stretch			
Aerobics/Anaerobics			
Weight Training			
Cross Training			
Cool Down			

ACTIVITY	EXERCISE	MIN/REPS	NOTES
Warm-Up			
Stretch			
Aerobics/Anaerobics			
Weight Training			
Power Training			
Cross Training			
Cool Down			

SKIERS' RESPONSIBILITY CODE

Like any other sport, skiing has its inherent risks and dangers. However, every year there are many injuries that can easily be avoided if we all take responsibility for our actions and the way we ski. Please take the time to learn the SKIERS' RESPONSIBILITY CODE and put it to use on the slopes.

1) Ski in control so that you can stop or avoid other skiers or objects.

2) When skiing downhill or overtaking another skier, you must avoid the skier below you.

3) Do not stop where you obstruct a trail or are not visible from above.

4) When entering a trail or starting downhill, yield to other skiers.

5) All skiers must wear retention straps or other devices to prevent runaway skis.

6) Keep off closed trails and posted areas and observe all posted signs.

SKI SHAPE:

How To Get Fit For Skiing....

The perfect gift for your friends, customers and business associates.

To order more copies of Ski Shape: How To Get Fit For Skiing simply fill out the coupon below (photo copies are o.k.) and send it along with a check or money order or call 1-800-444-2524 ext 67 (all major credit cards are accepted)

Send $12.95 per book plus $3.25 for shipping and handling

Send order and payment to:
PIONEER BOOKS, INC
5715 N. Balsam Road
Las Vegas, Nevada 89130

NAME:_____

STREET:_____

CITY:_____

STATE/ZIP:_____

TOTAL:_____ SHIPPING:_____

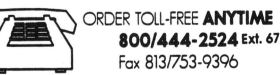

ORDER TOLL-FREE **ANYTIME**
800/444-2524 Ext. 67
Fax 813/753-9396

Here's a few Pioneer books to read while you're in the jacuzzi at the end of your ski day. . . .

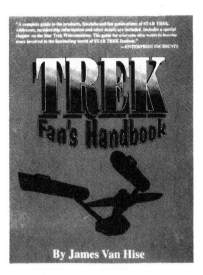

THE TREK FAN'S HANDBOOK

Written by James Van Hise

STAR TREK inspired its millions of loyal fans to put pen to paper, in order to discuss the various themes and issues being raised by the show's scripts, explore the characters in minute detail and ponder where both STAR TREK and humanity are headed in the future.

THE TREK FAN'S HANDBOOK offers a guide on who to write to, what products are available, information on the various STAR TREK fanclubs, addresses, membership information and details on the fanzines they publish.

THE TREK FAN'S HANDBOOK allows the reader to tap into the basic backbone of what has allowed STAR TREK to thrive over the past quarter century.

$9.95 ISBN#1-55698- 271-2

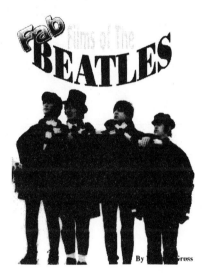

THE FAB FILMS OF THE BEATLES

Written by Edward Gross

The phenomenon of the Beatles began in 1964 and has become legend. Their films (A HARD DAY'S NIGHT, HELP, MAGICAL MYSTERY TOUR, YELLOW SUBMARINE and LET IT BE) are movie classics. A HARD DAY'S NIGHT revolutionized the rock film.

THE FAB FILMS OF THE BEATLES provides an in-depth examination of the Beatles films and motion pictures about them, going behind the scenes of each and presenting profiles of the Beatles themselves, synopsis, commentary, a look at their impact and side-bar features. In addition, the book looks at the solo film efforts of John Lennon, Paul McCartney, George Harrison and Ringo Starr, including Lennon's HOW I WON THE WAR, McCartney's GIVE MY REGARDS TO BROAD STREET, Harrison's various Handmade Films and Starr's CAVEMAN. Also, for the first time anywhere, the text provides a comprehensive guide to the group and solo music videos, an integral aspect of their filmmaking career.

$14.95 ISBN # 1-55698-244-5

FORTY YEARS AT NIGHT

The Tonight Show Story

Scott Nance

• In May 1992, Johnny Carson will retire and hand over "The Tonight Show" mike to comedian Jay Leno

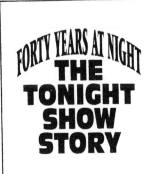

"The Tonight Show" began as a local variety show in the early 1950s and eventually established itself as a piece of American culture. This entertaining book chronicles the show's 40-year history and gives behind-the-scenes views through the eyes of Ed McMahon, Doc Severinsen, executive producer Fred de Cordova, as well as many of the stars who have appeared throughout the years.

Scott Nance writes for a variety of entertainment magazines and is the author of *ZZ Top: Recycling the Blues.*

$14.95, Trade paper, ISBN 1-55698-308-5

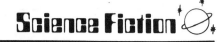

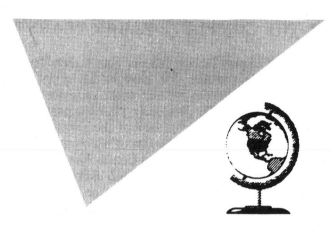

The Lost In Space Technical Manual, featuring technical diagrams to all of the spacecraft and devices, as well as exclusive production artwork.

Limited Edition: $14.95

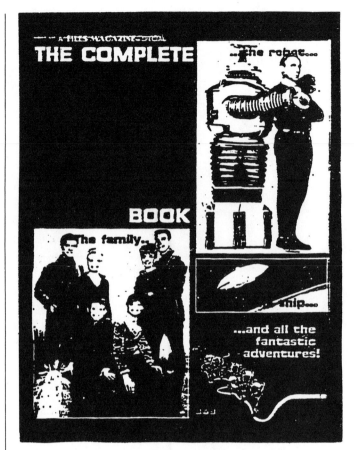

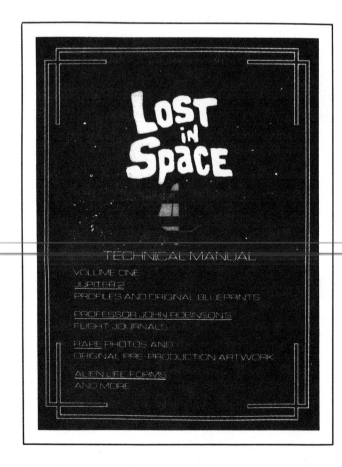

THE COMPLETE LOST IN SPACE
Written by John Peel

The complete guide to every single episode of LOST IN SPACE including profiles of every cast member and character.

The most exhaustive book ever written about LOST IN SPACE.

$19.95...220 pages

Couch Potato Inc.   5715 N. Balsam   Las Vegas, NV 89130   (702)658-2090

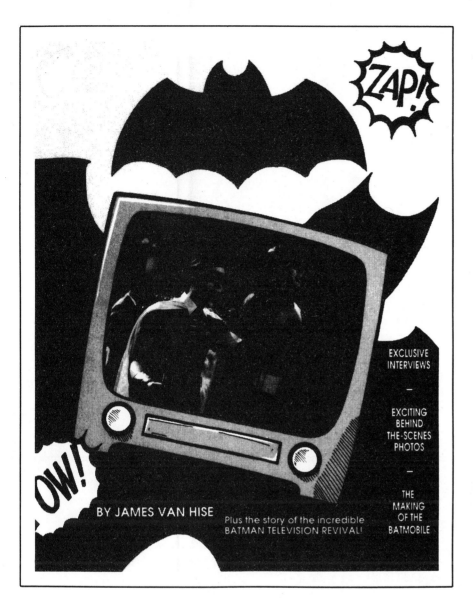

BATMANIA II
Written by James Van Hise

Available in June.
Updating BATMANIA to include coverage of the second movie plus additional new material.
$14.95
.Color cover,
black and white interior photos
ISBN#1-55698-315-8

BATMANIA
(3rd printing) Written by James Van Hise
Tracing the Batman phenomenon over the past 50 years, beginning with the character's creation by Bob Kane in 1939, and examining the changes in the pages of Detective Comics and his own title over the last five decades. Then the focus shifts to the two movie serials and jumps two decades to the enormously popular BATMAN television series of the 1960s, the primary focus of the book. Interviews with Adam West (Batman), Burt Ward (Robin), Yvonne Craig (Batgirl), Julie Newmar (The Catwoman), writer Stanley Ralph Ross and George Barris, who designed the various Bat-vehicles, bring the reader behind the scenes. Special sections showcase the innumerable collectibles inspired by the show, and the ongoing phenomenon that surrounds it.
BATMANIA is the ultimate Bat-book for Bat-fans!
$14.95..........164 pages Color Cover, Black and White Interior Photos
ISBN#1-55698-252-6

Couch Potato Inc.   5715 N. Balsam   Las Vegas, NV 89130   (702)658-2090

Boring, But Necessary Ordering Information!

Payment:
> All orders must be prepaid by check or money order. Do not send cash. All payments must be made in US funds only.

Shipping:
> We offer several methods of shipment for our product. Sometimes a book can be delayed if we are temporarily out of stock. You should note on your order whether you prefer us to ship the book as soon as available or send you a merchandise credit good for other goodies or send you your money back immediately.

Postage is as follows:

Normal Post Office: For books priced under $10.00—for the first book add $2.50. For each additional book under $10.00 add $1.00. (This is per indidividual book priced under $10.00. Not the order total.) For books priced over $10.00—for the first book add $3.25. For each additional book over $10.00 add $2.00.(This is per individual book priced over $10.00, not the order total.) These orders are filled as quickly as possible. Shipments normally take 2 or 3 weeks, but allow up to 12 weeks for delivery.

Special UPS 2 Day Blue Label Rush Service or Priority Mail(Our Choice). Special service is available for desperate Couch Potatoes. These books are shipped within 24 hours of when we receive the order and should normally take 2 to 3 days to get from us to you.

For the first RUSH SERVICE book under $10.00 add $5.00. For each additional 1 book under $10.00 add $1.75. (This is per individual book priced under $10.00, not the order total.)

For the first RUSH SERVICE book over $10.00 add $7.00 For each additional book over $10.00 add $4.00 per book.(This is per individual book priced over $10.00, not the order total.)

Canadian shipping rates add 20% to the postage total.

Foreign shipping rates add 50% to the postage total.
> All Canadian and foreign orders are shipped either book or printed matter.
> Rush Service is not available.

DISCOUNTS!DISCOUNTS!
> Because your orders keep us in business we offer a discount to people that buy a lot of our books as our way of saying thanks. On orders over $25.00 we give a 5% discount. On orders over $50.00 we give a 10% discount. On orders over $100.00 we give a 15% discount. On orders over over $150.00 we giver a 20 % discount.

Please list alternates when possible.

Please state if you wish a refund or for us to backorder an item if it is not in stock.

100% satisfaction guaranteed.
> We value your support. You will receive a full refund as long as the copy of the book you are not happy with is received back by us in reasonable condition. No questions asked, except we would like to know how we failed you. Refunds and credits are given as soon as we receive back the item you do not want.

Please have mercy on Phyllis and carefully fill out this form in the neatest way you can. Remember, she has to read a lot of them every day and she wants to get it right and keep you happy! You may use a duplicate of this order blank as long as it is clear. Please don't forget to include payment! And remember, we love repeat friends.

_____Trek: The Lost Years $12.95   ISBN#1-55698-220-8

_____Trek: The Next Generation $14.95   ISBN#1-55698-305-0

_____Trek: Twentyfifth Anniversary Celebration $14.95   ISBN#1-55698-290-9

_____The Making Of The Next Generation $14.95   ISBN#1-55698-219-4

_____The Best Of Enterprise Incidents: The Mag For Star Trek Fans $9.95 ISBN#1-55698-231-3

_____The History Of Trek $14.95   ISBN#1-55698-309-3

_____Trek Fan's Handbook $9.95   ISBN#1-55698-271-2

_____The Trek Crewbook $9.95   ISBN#1-55698-257-7

_____The Man Between The Ears: Star Trek's Leonard Nimoy $14.95   ISBN#1-55698-304-2

_____The Doctor And The Enterprise $9.95   ISBN#1-55698-218-6

_____The Lost In Space Tribute Book $14.95   ISBN#1-55698-226-7

_____The Complete Lost In Space $19.95

_____The Lost In Space Tech Manual $14.95

_____Doctor Who: The Complete Baker Years $19.95   ISBN#1-55698-147-3

_____The Doctor Who Encyclopedia: The Baker Years $19.95 ISBN#1-55698-160-0

_____Doctor Who: The Pertwee Years $19.95   ISBN#1-55698-212-7

_____Number Six: The Prisoner Book $14.95   ISBN#1-55698-158-9

_____Gerry Anderson: Supermarionation $14.95

_____The L.A. Lawbook $14.95   ISBN#1-55698-295-X

_____The Rockford Phile $14.95   ISBN#1-55698-288-7

_____Cheers: Where Everybody Knows Your Name $14.95   ISBN#1-55698-291-7

_____It's A Bird It's A Plane $14.95   ISBN#1-55698-201-1

_____The Green Hornet Book $16.95 Edition

_____How To Draw Art For Comic Books $14.95   ISBN#1-55698-254-2

_____How To Create Animation $14.95   ISBN#1-55698-285-2

_____Rocky & The Films Of Stallone $14.95   ISBN#1-55698-225-9

_____The New Kids Block $9.95   ISBN#1-55698-242-9

_____Monsterland Fearbook $14.95

_____The Unofficial Tale Of Beauty And The Beast $14.95   ISBN#1-55698-261-5

_____The Hollywood Death Book $14.95   ISBN#1-55698-307-7

_____The Addams Family Revealed $14.95   ISBN#1-55698-300-X

_____The Dark Shadows Tribute Book $14.95   ISBN#1-55698-234-8

_____Stephen King & Clive Barker: An Illustrated Guide $14.95 ISBN#1-55698-253-4

_____Stephen King & Clive Barker: Illustrated Guide II $14.95 ISBN#1-55698-310-7

_____The Fab Films Of The Beatles $14.95   ISBN#1-55698-244-5

_____Paul McCartney: 20 Years On His Own $9.95   ISBN#1-55698-263-1

_____Yesterday: My Life With the Beatles $14.95   ISBN#1-55698-292-5

_____Forty Years At Night: The Tonight Show Story   ISBN#1-55698-308-5 $14.95

_____The Films Of Elvis: The Magic Lives On $14.95   ISBN#1-55698-223-2

_____Batmania $14.95   ISBN#1-55698-252-6

_____Batmania II $14.95   ISBN#1-55698-315-8

_____The Phantom Serials $16.95

_____Batman Serials $16.95

_____Batman & Robin Serials $16.95

_____The Complete Batman & Robin Serials $19.95

_____The Green Hornet Serials $16.95

_____The Flash Gordon Serials Part 1 $16.95

_____The Flash Gordon Serials Part 2 $16.95

_____The Shadow Serials $16.95

_____Blackhawk Serials $16.95

_____Serial Adventures $14.95   ISBN#1-55698-236-4

_____Encyclopedia Of Cartoon Superstars $14.95   ISBN#1-55698-269-0

_____The Woody Allen Encyclopedia $14.95   ISBN#1-55698-303-4

_____The Gunsmoke Years $14.95   ISBN#1-55698-221-6

_____The Wild Wild West $14.95   ISBN#1-55698-162-7

_____Who Was That Masked Man $14.95   ISBN#1-55698-227-5

_____The Man Who Created Star Trek $14.95   ISBN #1-55698-318-2

_____Trek: The Making of the Movies $14.95   ISBN#1-55698-313-1

NAME:_____

STREET:_____

CITY:_____

STATE:_____

ZIP:_____

TOTAL:_____ SHIPPING_____

SEND TO: Couch Potato, Inc. 5715 N. Balsam Rd., Las Vegas, NV 89130